CONTENTS

For many years I have been so inspired by so many teachers. From my first baby step into the mad world of Kundalini, when my gorgeous cousin grabbed me in Los Angeles, when she was working on American Idol and threw me into a workshop with Gurmukh.

To be introduced to Yogi Tea, to monks who just travel and visit people, to learning about the in-depth work that Kundalini does to each chakra. To learning from Patricia Grube, Maya Fiennes, Gurmukh and to following the perfect teachings of Yogi Bhajan.

*This book is my Yorkshire Yoga version of Kundalini, I may never travel to Los Angeles again. I may never meet these people again. Our lives take so many twists and turns. This book in a series brings together the 7 wonderful chakras and allows **you** to work on each one, one at a time.*

*My first **Crystal Clear** works on Chakra 1, my second **Inspiring Yourself and Others** works on Chakra 2.*

I look forward to bringing more Chakras to our Yogi Playground. Ones you can do at home be you a yoga teacher, a yogi, or just interested in learning a little bit more about Yoga and in particular Kundalini Yoga. Welcome to this wonderful World!

I dedicate this book to my teachers, my family and my friends, our brilliant yoga community, my amazing, patient, husband, my beautiful children and. of course, Rosie the dog.

BECOMING
Crystal Clear

MULADHARA: THE FIRST CHAKRA

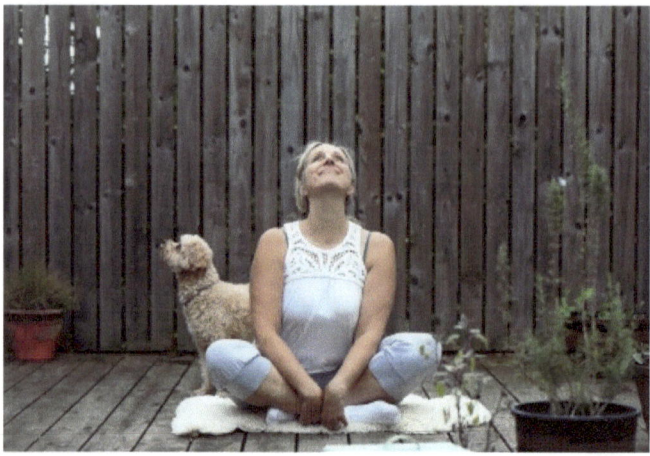

This chakra is about survival, the urge to exist here on this planet. If you fail to survive you die so this drive is extremely powerful. This chakra is linked to the adrenal glands and the fight or flight instinct. It is responsible for strength and stability, grounding, financial worth, material worth, your home, your castle, your neighbourhood.

An imbalanced chakra comes from early years with upheaval, with being passed from one person to the next and thus not bonding fully with carers. Imbalance can activate later in life with a fall or damage (especially if the perineum is damaged during childbirth).

The lower chakras are very important for the whole ascent and descent of energy through the Ida and Pingala system and a strong base chakra is essential.

The first chakra

is known as

'the base chakra'

COLOUR- RED

Sound – Lam

Location – Base of Pelvis

Image (Yantra) – Four Lotus Petals
Affirmation – "I exist"
Element – Earth
Kosha – Annamayakosha
**Traditional Postures – Standing poses like Mountain, Triangle. Hip openers like Bound Angle and Frog.
Associated with the pelvis, legs and feet and
all aspects of elimination.**

Musical Note- C
Solfeggio Frequency – 396 Hz
Sense - Smell
Essential Oils - Patchouli, cypress, myrrh, vetiver
**Crystals - Garnet, Obsidian, Ruby, Red Jasper,
Haematite, Smoky Quartz**

Physical Problems related to the chakra include -

Infections of the urinary system, poor teeth and/or bones, stiff or painful lower back, sciatica, hip issues, problems in the lower digestive tract, piles and inflammatory bowel disease, skin problems, lack of energy.

Key words -
*Acceptance, stability, self-preservation, being
grounded, fear and safety.*

THE FIRST CHAKRA AND THE GLANDS

The first chakra, is associated with male gonads the testes as well as the adrenal glands. Ruling the bowel, anus, legs and feet, lower back, perineum, colon, urethra tubes, bladder, hips and male and female reproductive organs.

First Chakra Warm Up
Spinal Flex

Sit in easy pose and hold the ankles, with both hands, deeply inhale as you flex the spine forward. Open the chest and the shoulders. On the exhale, flex the spine backwards. Keeping the head parallel to the ground so it doesn't flip flop.

Inhale forwards exhale backwards
Synchronise the breath for 2 minutes

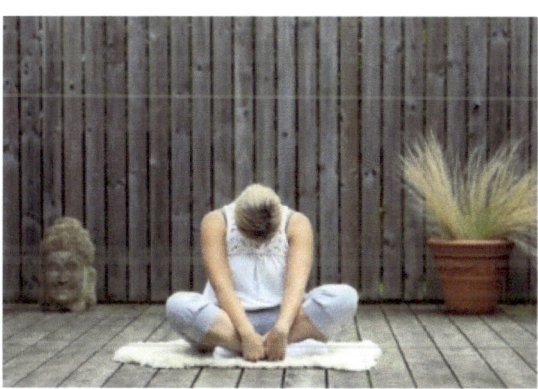

Sophie Bickerdike

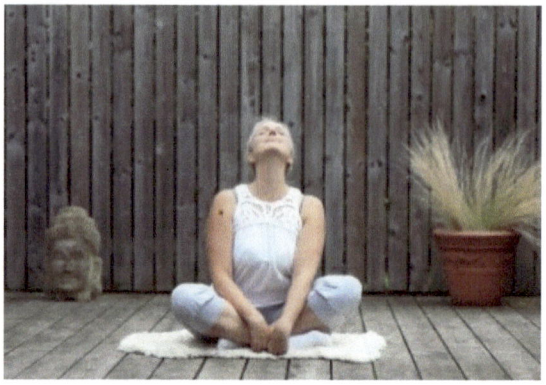

SUFIS GRIND

Grasp the knees firmly and circle the spine round. The spine is a spoon, the pelvis is a bowl, you are stirring the bowl with your spine. Warming up the base chakra and the lower chakras. Grind for 2 minutes

Finish and engage Mulabandha, navel in, keep squeezing the sex organs, anus for 20 seconds….. (did I really just write that!), make sure your shoulders are relaxed.

You are awakening the Kundalini now!

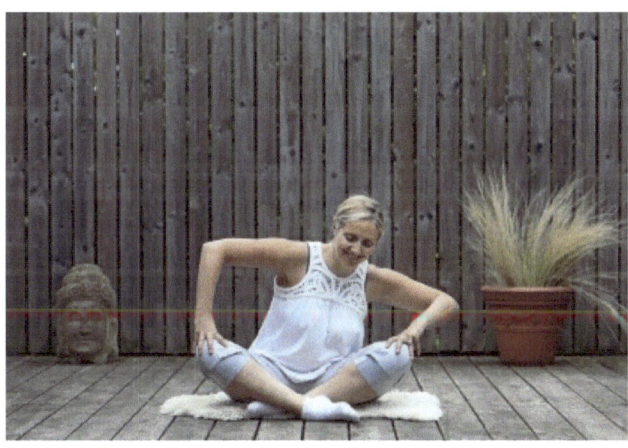

Sophie Bickerdike

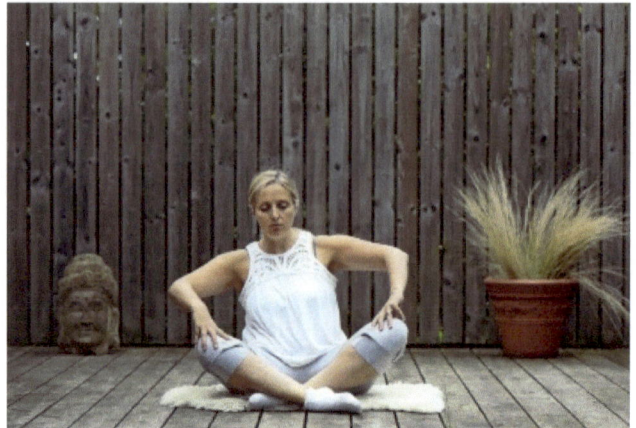

NECK ROLLS

Bring the index fingers to the thumbs sitting cross-legged palms up. This activates the Jupiter energy. Your index finger is Jupiter and your thumb is the earth. When your index finger touches the thumb you receive inner knowledge.

Relax for 30 seconds.

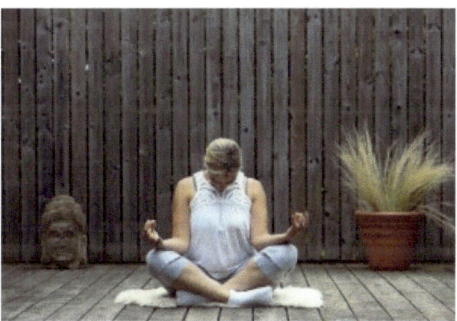

Hold your shoulders and twist to the left inhale, exhale and twist to the right. You are keeping the elbows high, arms parallel to the ground. Keep on!

Inhale, exhale.

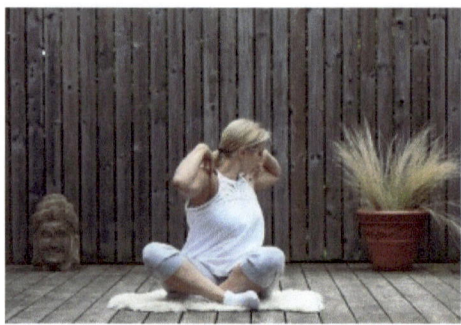

Roll the neck clockwise one minute in each direction.
Rotate the shoulders forwards in one direction and
backwards in the other direction.

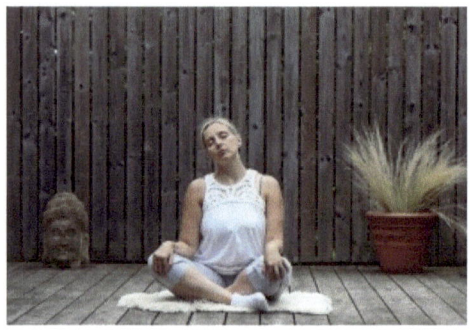

LIFE NERVE STRETCH

With legs stretched apart. Reach up and stretch along one leg inhale then lift up and reach along the other leg, exhale... Continue for 2 minutes.

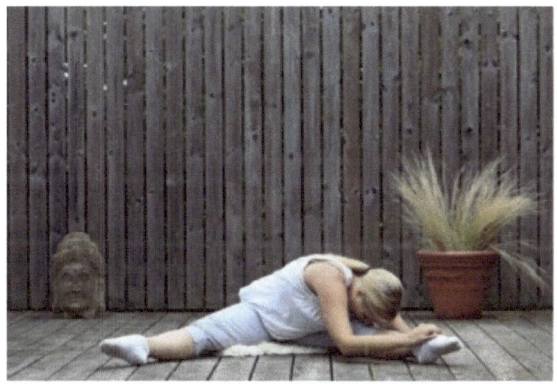

Once relaxed sit in gyan mudra.

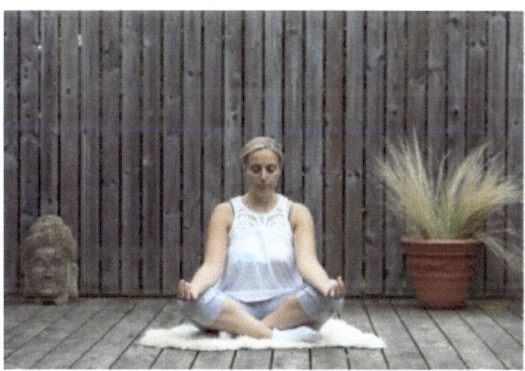

FIRST CHAKRA KRIYA

Sit on your left heel. Put hands on floor by your hips. Breathe in deeply, and as you breathe out lean forwards. Breathe in as you come back up and continue this movement. Watch your breath. Continue for 2 minutes.

Repeat the same exercise but now with both legs out. Continue for 2 minutes.

LIE BACK AND RELAX. Inhale and hold bring the knees to the chest. Breathe in and out and RELAX.

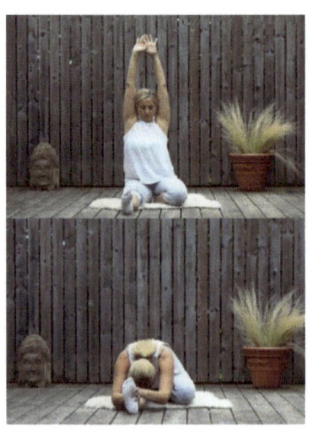

LIE BACK

Stretch out your legs, breathe in deeply, and you breathe out sit upright, lean forwards and grab your toes. Breathe in and lie down again. Mentally vibrate Sat as you breathe in and Nam as you breathe out.

Inhale and exhale.

Continue for 2 minutes.

Use your abdominals to protect your spine.

As an expansion to this...

Rock right back into plough/Halasana.

Inhale to legs over your head and exhale to forward bend.

Continue for a further 2 minutes.

Once finished knees come into the chest to release the lower back.

Relax.

Sophie Bickerdike

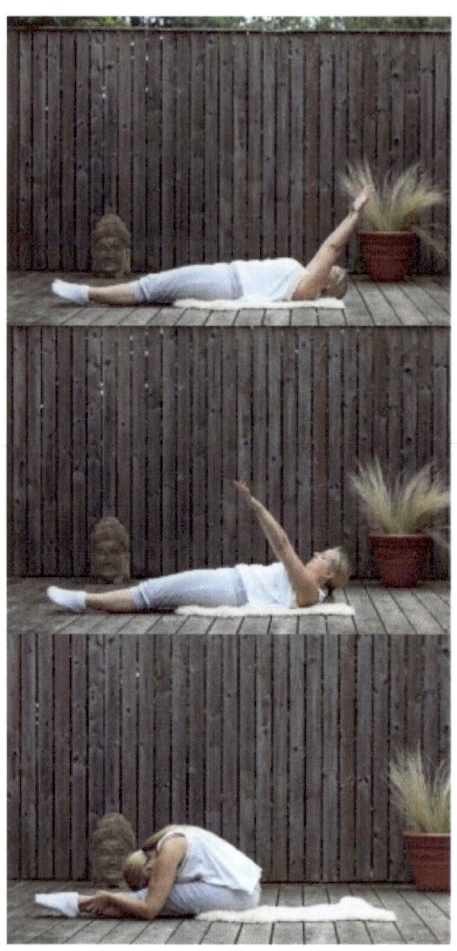

SQUAT IN FROG POSE

Squat with toes turned out heels kissing. Fingertips to floor, eyes closed and focus your attention on the third eye. Look in-between your eyebrows. Breathe in and straighten your legs, raise your hips up, keeping your hands on the ground. Heels remain lifted.

Breathe out and return to squat.
Repeat 26 times.

This is good for the prevention of breast and prostate cancer as it raises the energy from the lower to the higher centres.

On completion come up place hands on hips and breathe in through the nose and out of the mouth five times.To finish sit in easy pose cross-legged.

"The energy of the universe is yours.
It is your birth-right. Just claim it."

Yogi Bhajan

Sophie Bickerdike

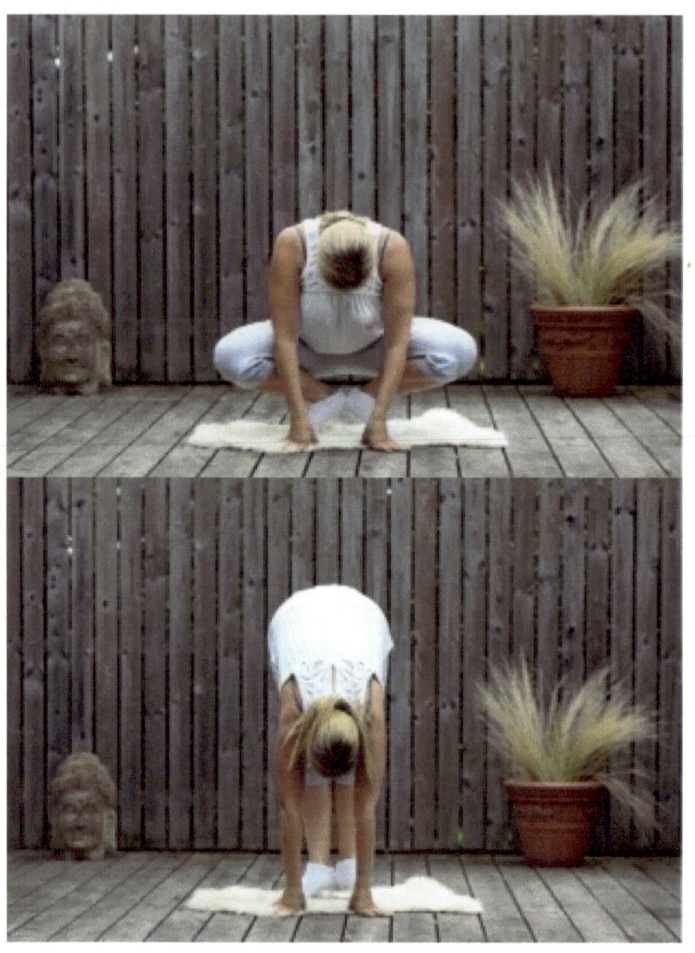

FURTHER CROW POSE

With your feet shoulder distance apart, you can place two chairs beside you for support, try to squat. If you can't get right down straight down and can go only half way, go down onto the balls of the feet, and slowly move inch by inch. Once you reach as far you can go down, extend your arms out in front and stretch your index fingers out straight in front of you, as if you were pointing towards some distant spot in front of you.

Keep your eyes one tenth open, extend your tongue and begin panting through the open mouth as you pump your belly in and out along with the breath, like a dog. Begin with one minute and build up to 3 minutes.

Relax again in easy pose.

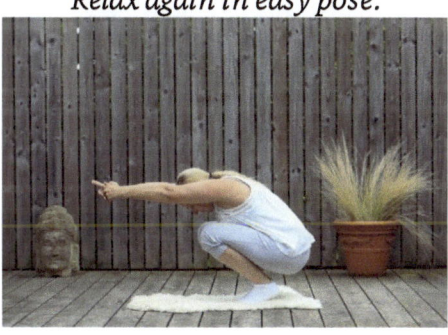

FIRST CHAKRA MEDITATION FOR REJUVENATION

Sit in easy pose and interlace the fingers with the thumbs unlocked and touching at the tips. Apply root lock, pulling the end of the colon, sexual organs up tightly, keep this contraction and chant "God and me, me and God are one" or alternately "Wahe Guru Wahe Guru"

Exhale, release the contractions. Inhale deeply and repeat.

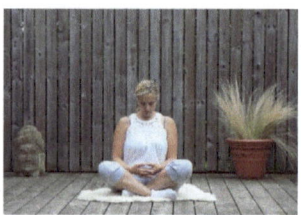

"If a person can apply root lock, he becomes invincible." **Yogi Bhajan**

"Without Forgiveness, Life is Governed by an Endless Cycle of Resentment and Retaliation." **Robert Assagioli**

So, repeat the First Chakra exercises and meditation for 40 days. Journal as you go and only then move onto the Second Chakra.

INSPIRING YOURSELF
& Others

SVADHISTANA: THE SECOND CHAKRA

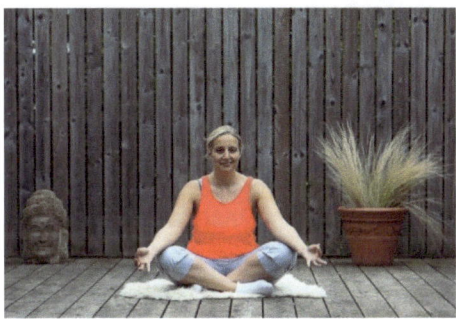

Through the Second Chakra you meet the world and the people who live in it. It is associated with wealth and creating money, allowing this chakra to flow, allows money to flow to and from you and back again. Repeat the following exercises for 40 days and note what happens. I suggest journalling as you go too and see what flows to you! These exercises are pretty wierd and wonderful so prepare yourself for change.

*(Some say this chakra is also associated with **guilt, feeling "less than"**.*

*Many surveys state most people's problems arise from issues around **money and love**...so this can be seen as an extra-important chakra!)*

COLOUR - ORANGE

Sound – Vam

**Location – Low Down in the Abdomen, just above the top
of the pubic bone, not far above the base chakra.**

Image (Yantra) – Six Lotus Petals
Affirmation – "I create"
Element – Water
Kosha – Pranamayakosha
**Traditional Postures – Baddha Konasana, eagle,
squats, balancing postures.**
**Associated with the pelvis, sexual organs, lower
vertebrae, kidneys, bladder, appendix, digestions, hip
area, lymphatic system, bodily fluids.**

Musical Note- D and C Sharp
Solfeggio Frequence – 417 Hz
Sense - Taste
Oils - Orange, tangerine, rosemary, juniper.
Crystals: Carnelian, coral, citrine, orange calcite and amber.

Physical Problems related to the chakra include -
*infertility, problems with the reproductive organs, allergies,
prostrate problems, sciatica, hip problems, urine infections, loss
of appetite for food and sex. Weak bladder and kidneys.*

Key words

Creativity and pleasure, finances, flow, emotions, addiction, creativity, change and movement.

SECOND CHAKRA
KRIYA

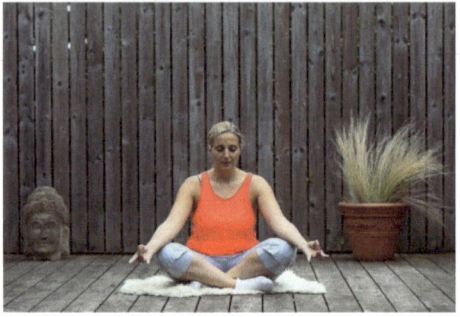

Breath meditation to regulate hormones, male or female.

(especially good for the menstrual cycle and prostrate issues)

Sit in easy pose and press the index finger to the thumb
on the first sniff, mentally vibrate **SAA.**
Press the middle finger to the thumb on the second sniff, mentally vibrate **TAA.**
Press the ring finger to the thumb on the third
sniff, mentally vibrate **NAA.**
Press the little finger to the thumb on the fourth
sniff, mentally vibrate **MAA.**

Exhale in one long stroke.

The rhythm will be 8 beats, inhale segmented breath in 4
strokes and exhale in one long stroke for 4 beats.
(Eyes closed)

(On a physical level, the pituitary gland and pineal glands are stimulated and brought into rhythm by the four part breathing. On a mental level, thought patterns can be erased and a new balance established. On an auric level, a clear radiance and projection can be achieved.)

BALANCING CREATIVE ENERGY

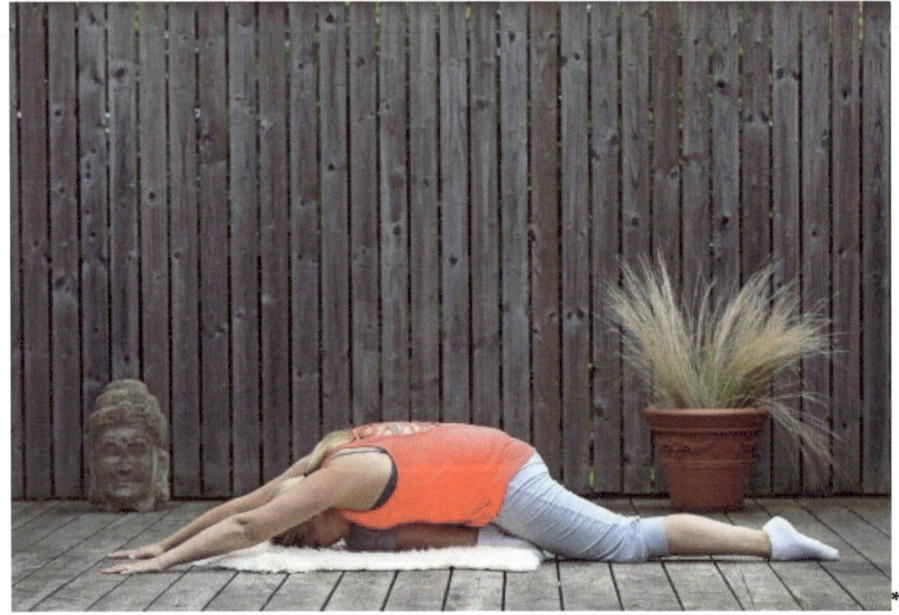

Sit on the heels. Extend the left leg straight back along the ground. Bend forward and place the forehead on the ground.

Put both arms back along the sides, palms upwards. Relaxing all the muscles and breathe slowly and deeply for 3 minutes. You then slowly come up on the inhale, and repeat on the other side for a further 3 minutes.

Gradually increase the time to 11 minutes.

(The pituitary gland is stimulated and the ovaries/gonads are relaxed. This is also good for the eyes.)

EAR MASSAGE

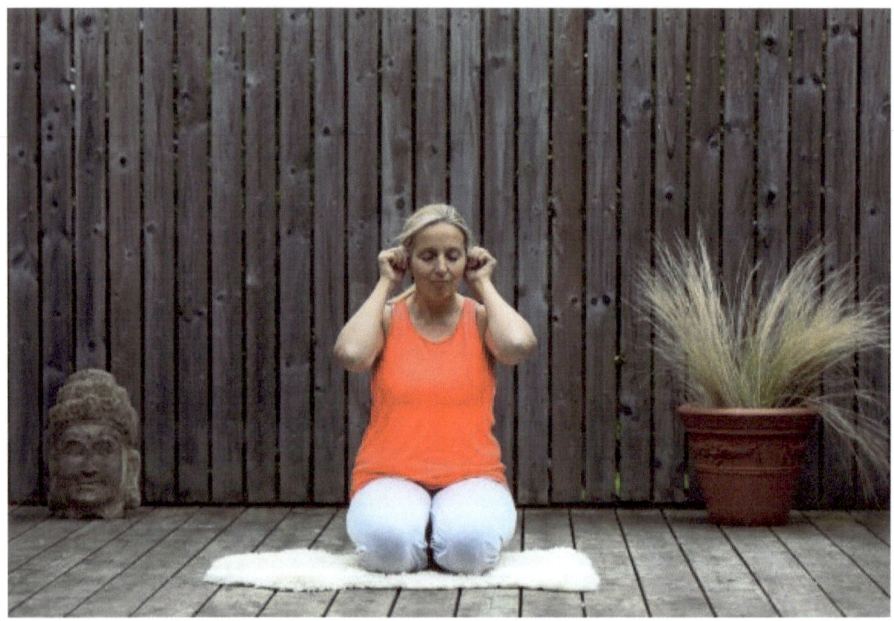

Still on the heels. Bring the heel of the hands to the ears, keeping the fingers together and pointed slightly behind you. Create a slight angle at the wrists so the fingers point away from the skull.

Massage the ears and earlobes with the palms.

Alternate between circular motion and

linear up and down strokes.

Continue for 2-3 minutes. Inhale and gently pull the earlobes downward and away from the body. Hold for 10 seconds and relax.

(There are meridian points on the ears that govern all parts of the body. It is massaging the whole body using just the ears. You will feel the blood flow come into the ears and you will feel much more balanced and warm.)

FRONT LOCUST LIFT

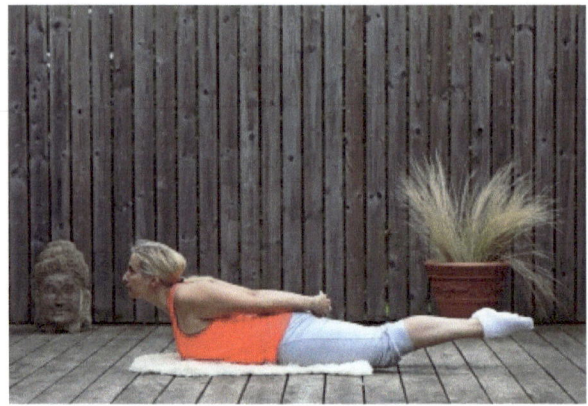

Lying on your front with your fingers interlaced behind.
Breathe in and lift legs and arms keeping your knees
and elbows straight. Start breath of Fire.

Continue for 3 minutes.

(This strengthens the reproductive organs,
digestive system and abdominals.)

TORSO TWISTS

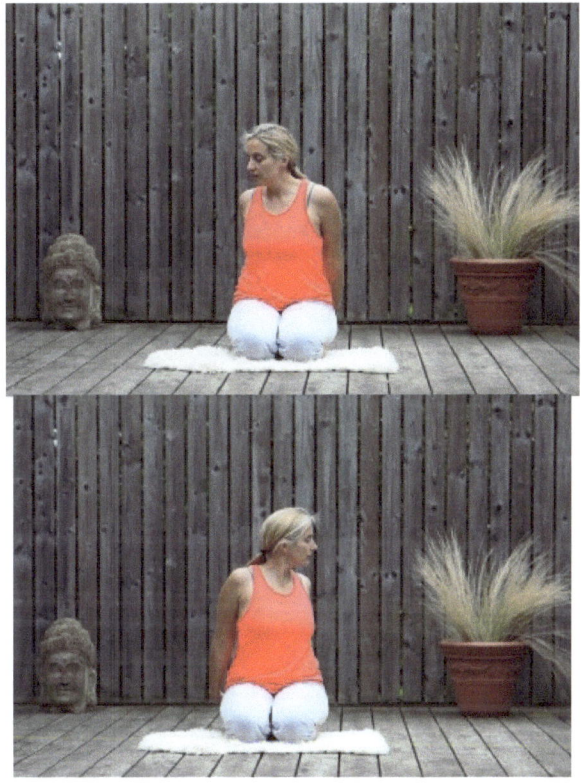

Still sitting on the heels, immediately interlace the fingers in Venus Lock at the base of the spine.

Keep the spine straight. Inhale deeply as you twist the torso to the left. Exhale and turn to the right.

The motion is moderately slow and complete.

Continue for 3 minutes.

To end inhale, pull mulabandha in and lengthen the spine. See the energy flowing up the centre of the spine rejuvenating and relaxing the whole body.

Inhale and exhale.

(This helps elimination and is good for the lumbar spine.)

SIT-UPS MAKING LEGS WIDE

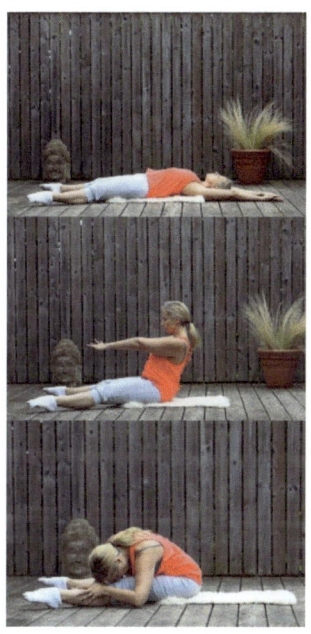

Lie on the back. Spread the legs as wide as possible, without strain. Grasp the shoulders and let the elbows rest on the ground – if this is too much reach the arms in front. Hold this position for 3 minutes. Inhale deeply as you lie back and relax.

Gradually rise up and forward again.

This time bend over the left knee. Hold for one minute. Inhale, then exhale deeply 3 times. Then inhale deeply as you lie back. Repeat the same sit up and hold over the right leg. Hold for 1 minute. Inhale and exhale deeply 3 times.

Then inhale deeply as you lie back.

(This works on the sciatic nerve and its branches round the back of the chakra. It strengthens the abdomen and releases tension caused by anxiety.)

KNEE AND ELBOW WALK

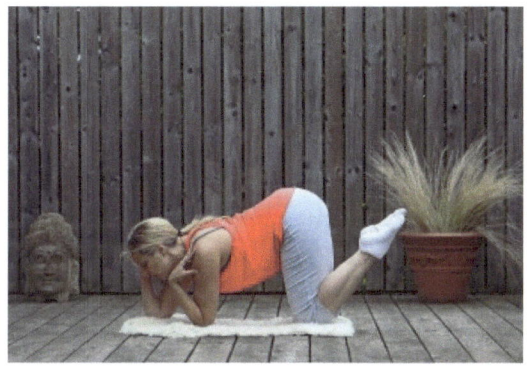

Balance on the hands and knees. Raise the heels towards the buttocks. Place the elbows on the ground, with the hands up by the shoulders. Raise the head so you can see forward. Begin to walk on elbows and knees.

Continue for 3 minutes.

Relax completely for 1 minute.

(This promotes circulation, works on the heart and improves mineral balance.)

LOTUS WALK

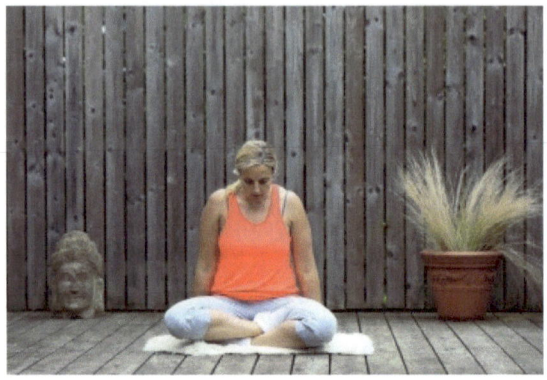

Sitting in full half or simply cross-legged. Lean forward onto hands. Try and lift up the body and swing it forward. Try and move along the ground.

Try and move for 3 minutes.

(This opens the navel point energy and

rebalances the sex organs).

BACK PLATFORM POSE

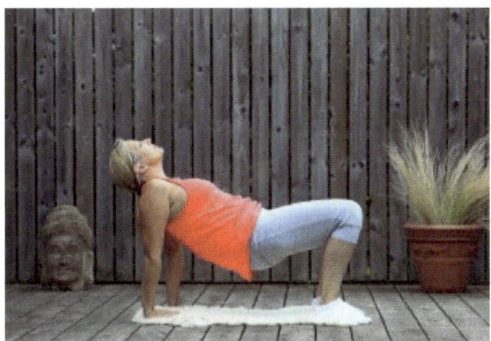

Sit straight with the legs stretched, put the hands on the ground by the hips and lift the legs, hips and chest up to form a platform from the chin to the toes.

Begin to walk on the heels and hands.

Continue for three minutes.

Relax totally for 15 minutes, feeling weight-less and floating in orange ethers.

(This energy releases tension in the sex meridians. It enhances circulation in the pelvic region and activates the second chakra and all its sources.)

SECOND CHAKRA MEDITATION

LONG EK ONG KAR

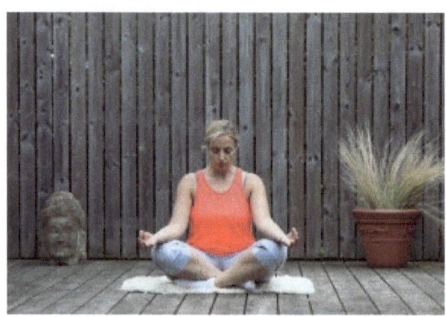

"This mantra is used as the cornerstone of morning sadhana, it initiates the relationships of the soul with the universal soul. It balances all of the chakras. All mantras are good, and are for the awakening of the Divine. But this mantra is effective, and is the mantra for this Era. So my lovely student, at the will of my Master I teach you the greatest Divine key. It has eight levers, and can open the lock of the time, which is also the vibration of the eight. Therefore, when this mantra is chanted with the Neck Lock, at the point where prana and apana meet sushumuna, this vibration opens the lock, and thus one becomes one with the Divine." **Yogi Bhajan**

How to perform LONG EK ONG KAR WITH NECK LOCK

Sit in easy pose with a firm neck lock.

Have the hands in Gyan Mudra, or resting on the knees in Buddha Mudra. Maintain a strong neck lock. We are going to activate the reproductive organs with this mantra.

Chant EK pulling in the navel in abruptly.

Then release with ONG KAAR. Inhale deeply pull in the navel abruptly, chant SAT, then NAAM out.

Inhale a half breath,

Pull in the navel

abruptly and chant

"Whaa, hay guroo".

Keep the pitch the same. Let the sound resonate in the upper cavity of the head, by closing the back of the throat and vibrating the upper palate, and allowing the sound to come through the nose. Start with 3 minutes and build up to 11 minutes, 31 minutes or even 2 hours!

MORE ON THE SECOND CHAKRA

The Second Chakra, is associated with balancing the hormones and levels of oestrogen and testosterone in the body.

The Second Chakra can both invigorate and soothe the body with these practises.

As you journal note how this changes how your body feels before and after the practice.

After 40 days how do you feel?

Time to go to the third chakra.

The energy of Creation.

Join Me.

REFERENCES

Anatomy and Physiology in Health and Fitness 11th Edition, Ross and Wilson, Churchhill, Livingstone and Elsevier. Anne Waugh & Alison Grant, 2010.

Ashtanga Yoga: The Practice Manual, Swenson, David. 1-891252-08-9.

Charm City Yoga: Practice Manual.

Light on Yoga, BKS Iyengar; Thorsons 2001.

Yoga; Danielou, Alain; Inner Traditions International, Rochester, VT 1991.

The Heart of Yoga, Inner Traditions International, Rochester, VT 1995.

Encyclopaedic Dictionary of Yoga, Paragon House, New York, NY, 1995; Feuerstein, Georg.

Living Yoga, The Putnum Publishing Group, New York, NY, 1993; Feuerstein, Georg and Bodian, Stephen.

Ashtanga Yoga Video, Delphi Productions, Boulder, CO,1993; Freeman, Richard.

Asana, The Sky Foundation, Philadelphia, PA 1978; Kuvalyananada, Swami
Pranayama, Bombay Popular, Prakasham, 1964; Kuvalayananda, Swami

Yoga for the Body, Rudra Press, Portland, OR, e International Association of Yoga Therapists, CA, 1993; Mohan, AG.

The Yoga of Understanding; Yogeshwarananda, Swami, CSA Press, Publishers, Lakemont, Georgie, 30552. (1986)

Bhagavad Gita,

Fiennes, Maya, Yoga for Real Life.

Cash, Mel, Pocket Atlas of the Moving Body, Ebury Press, 1999.

The Upanishads: A Selection from 108 Upanishads Hardcover – 1 Mar 2006 by T. M. P. Mahadevan (Editor), Bharatiya Kala Prakashan (Mar 2006)

Soul to Soul; Poems, Prayers and Stories to End a Yoga Class, Red Elixir Books, 2010; Mundahl, John.

Bailliere's Nurses Dictionary, Barbara F Weller; 1999 Harcourt Brace and Company, Bailliere Tindall published in association with RCN

The Human Body, Parker, Steve, 2007,DK.

Human Anatomy Coloring Book, Matt Margaret, Ziemian Joe, 1992 Dover Publications.

Key Muscles of Yoga

Ray Long

https://www.youtube.com/watch?v=fB6B9rQjEeU&spfreloa d=10

Jivamukti Work

http://jivamuktiyoga.com/category/content/mantra

Sophie Bickerdike

Likhita Mantra work
http://www.yasodhara.org/50th-anniversary-art-projects/likhita-japa/
The 8 Human Talents, Gurmukh with Cathryn Michon, 2000, by Narayan, LLC.
Anatomy and Physiology in Health and Wellness, Ross and Wilson, 11th Edition.
An Illustrated Guide to Every Part of the Human Body and How it Works, Ann
Baggeley.

DISCLAIMER

Not all exercises are suitable for everyone and this or any exercise programme may result in injury. To reduce the risk of injury, please follow the following guidelines.

Please eat your meal 1.5-2 hours before Yoga class. We recommend that this yoga is practised by those of 16 years and over. Please consult with a local yoga teacher before you commit to a practice. Always always practice in a safe and careful environment.

Avoid exerting yourself beyond capacity. Any pain or discomfort in a pose should be mild and temporary. Sharp and persistent pain is a sign of a physical problem or incorrect practice; consult your physician or yoga instructor.

Do not perform the inverted poses if you have high blood pressure, heart problems, detached retina or ear problems.

And always consult a medical practitioner before you begin your yoga practice.

Sophie Bickerdike a Yoga Elder with the Independent Yoga Network and Senior Yoga AllianceTeacher in the UK.
She runs GoYoga Studios and is co-creator of Go Revolution with Suzie Thomas. She trains Yoga Teachers and Primary Teachers to teach yoga and her dream with Helen Lehan is to bring yoga into schools nationwide.

Sophie Bickerdike

She has contributed to Bump and Beyond by Patricia Grube. Becoming and Inspiring is the first in her series of Chakra books.

www.ingramcontent.com/pod-product-compliance
Lightning Source LLC
Chambersburg PA
CBHW040327010626
45792CB00024B/2177